MW01519733

Ketogenic Recipes For Beginners

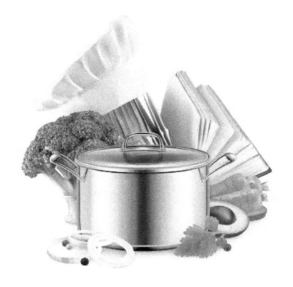

A Practical And Effective Guide To
Easy, Essential Fat Burning Recipes
For A Healthy Ketogenic Diet

Written By

Melissa Roberts

Table of Contents

INTRODUCTION

Thank you for purchasing this book!

Often these diets ask you to exercise more than five times a week. While this may seem like it is the way to go, the truth is that often people do not have the energy to do anything of the sort. This is not necessarily their fault. It is how they have lived and how they are living. That said, this new diet that does not require a calorie countdown or any sort of intellectual effort is the perfect match for people living that life. This diet does not care about calories, any fat content, what you eat or how you exercise.

Enjoy your reading!

BREAKFAST

Chicken Cheese Quiche

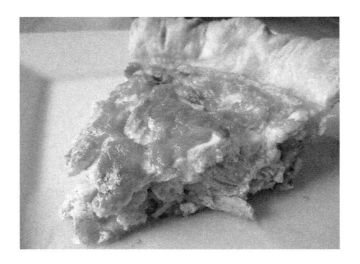

Level of difficulty: 5

Preparation time: 10 minutes

Servings: 4

Calories: 12 g

Condiments: Pepper and Salt

Protein: 19.2 g

Fat: 10 g

Ingredients:

- 8 eggs
- 1/2 tsp oregano
- 1/4 tsp onion powder
- 1/4 tsp garlic powder

- 1/4 cup mozzarella cheese, shredded
- 5 oz. cooked chicken breast, chopped
- 1/4 tsp pepper
- 1/2 tsp salt

Directions:

1. Preheat the oven to 350 F.
2. In a bowl, whisk eggs with oregano, onion powder, pepper, and salt. Stir in cheese and chicken.
3. Pour egg mixture in pie pan and bake for 35-45 minutes.
4. Slice and serve.

Turkey Cheese Frittata

Level of difficulty: 5

Preparation time: 10 minutes

Servings: 8

Calories: 1.2 g

Condiments: Salt and Pepper

Protein: 11.8 g

Fat: 6 g

Ingredients:

- 8 eggs
- 8 oz. turkey deli meat
- 2 tbsp. cheddar cheese, shredded
- 2 tbsp. parmesan cheese, shredded
- 1/2 tsp oregano
- 1/2 tsp thyme
- 1/4 tsp pepper
- 1/4 tsp salt

Directions:

1. Preheat the oven to 350 F.

2. Line an 8-inch skillet with the turkey deli meat.

3. In a bowl, whisk eggs with oregano, thyme, pepper, and salt. Pour egg mixture over meat.

4. Sprinkle parmesan cheese and cheddar cheese on top.

5. Bake for 20-25 minutes.

6. Serve and enjoy.

Swiss Chard Omelet

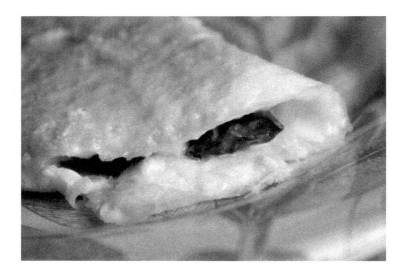

Level of difficulty: 5

Preparation time: 5 minutes

Servings: 2

Calories: 4 g

Condiments: Garlic Salt and Pepper

Protein: 14 g

Fat: 21 g

Ingredients:

- 2 eggs, lightly beaten
- 2 cups Swiss chard, sliced
- 1 tablespoon butter

- ½ teaspoon garlic salt
- Fresh pepper

Directions:

1. Take a non-stick frying pan and place it over medium-low heat.
2. Once the butter melts, add Swiss chard and stir cook for 2 minutes.
3. Pour egg into the pan and gently stir them into Swiss chard.
4. Season with garlic salt and pepper.
5. Cook for 2 minutes.
6. Serve and enjoy!

Coconut Porridge

Level of difficulty: 5

Preparation time: 15 minutes

Servings: 2

Calories: 5 g

Condiments: Protein Powder

Protein: 16 g

Fat: 13 g

Ingredients:

- 2 tablespoons coconut flour
- 2 tablespoons vanilla protein powder
- 3 tablespoons Golden Flaxseed Meal
- 1½ cups almond milk, unsweetened
- Powdered Erythritol

Directions:

1. Take a bowl, mix in flaxseed meal, protein powder, coconut flour, and mix well.
2. Add mix to a saucepan (placed over medium heat).
3. Add almond milk and stir, let the mixture thicken.
4. Add your desired amount of sweetener and serve.
5. Enjoy!

Scrambled Pesto Eggs

Level of difficulty: 5

Preparation time: 5 minutes

Servings: 2

Calories: 3 g

Condiments: Salt and Pepper

Protein: 20 g

Fat: 41 g

Ingredients:

- 2 large whole eggs
- 1/2 tablespoon butter
- 1/2 tablespoon pesto
- 1 tablespoon creamed coconut milk
- Salt, as needed
- pepper, as needed

Directions:

1. Take a bowl and crack open your egg.
2. Sprinkle with salt and pepper to your taste.
3. Pour eggs into a pan.
4. Add butter and introduce heat.

5. Cook on low heat and gently add pesto.

6. Once the egg is cooked and scrambled, remove heat.

7. Spoon in coconut cream and mix well.

8. Turn on the heat and cook on LOW for a while until you have a creamy texture.

9. Serve and enjoy!

Pepperoni Omelet

Level of difficulty: 5

Preparation time: 5 minutes

Servings: 2

Calories: 0.6 g

Condiments: Salt

Protein: 8.9 g

Fat: 11.5 g

Ingredients:

- 3 eggs
- 7 pepperoni slices
- 1 teaspoon coconut cream
- Salt
- freshly ground black pepper, to taste
- 1 tablespoons butter

Directions:

1. Take a bowl and whisk eggs with all the remaining Ingredients: in it.
2. Then take a skillet and heat butter.
3. Pour the ¼ of egg mixture into your skillet.

4. After that, cook for 2 minutes per side.

5. Repeat to use the entire batter.

6. Serve warm and enjoy!

Quinoa with Vegetables

Level of difficulty: 5

Preparation time: 10 minutes

Servings: 8

Calories: 204

Condiments: Salt and Pepper

Protein: 4 g

Fat: 3 g

Ingredients:

- 2 cups quinoa, rinsed and drained
- 2 onions, chopped
- 2 carrots, peeled and sliced
- 1 cup sliced cremini mushrooms
- 3 garlic cloves, minced
- 4 cups low-sodium vegetable broth
- 1/2 teaspoon salt
- 1 teaspoon dried marjoram leaves
- 1/8 teaspoon freshly ground black pepper

Directions:

1. In a 6-quart slow cooker, mix all of the ingredients.
2. Cover and cook on low for 5 to 6 hours, or until the quinoa and vegetables are tender.
3. Stir the mixture and serve.

MID MORNING

Coconut Kale Muffins

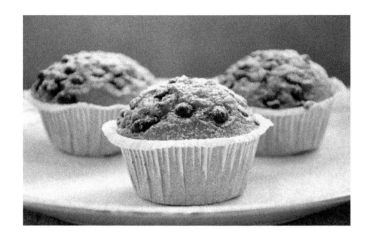

Level of difficulty: 5

Preparation time: 10 minutes

Servings: 8

Calories: 92

Condiments: Salt and Pepper

Protein: 5 g

Fat: 7 g

Ingredients:

- 6 eggs
- 1/2 cup unsweetened coconut milk
- 1 cup kale, chopped
- ¼ tsp garlic powder

26

- ¼ tsp paprika
- 1/4 cup green onion, chopped
- Pepper
- Salt

Directions:

1. Preheat the oven to 350 F.
2. Add all ingredients into the bowl and whisk well.
3. Pour mixture into the greased muffin tray and bake in oven for 30 minutes.
4. Serve and enjoy.

Protein Muffins

Level of difficulty: 5

Preparation time: 10 minutes

Servings: 12

Calories: 149

Condiments: Protein Powder

Protein: 8 g

Fat: 12 g

Ingredients:

- 8 eggs
- 2 scoop vanilla protein powder
- 8 oz. cream cheese
- 4 tbsp. butter, melted

Directions:

1. In a large bowl, combine cream cheese and melted butter.
2. Add eggs and protein powder and whisk until well combined.
3. Pour batter into the greased muffin pan.
4. Bake at 350 F for 25 minutes.
5. Serve and enjoy.

Healthy Waffles

Level of difficulty: 5

Preparation time: 10 minutes

Servings: 4

Calories: 220

Condiments: Stevia

Protein: 5.1 g

Fat: 17 g

Ingredients:

- 8 drops liquid stevia
- 1/2 tsp baking soda
- 1 tbsp. chia seeds
- 1/4 cup water
- 2 tbsp. sunflower seed butter
- 1 tsp cinnamon
- 1 avocado, peel, pitted and mashed
- 1 tsp vanilla
- 1 tbsp. lemon juice
- 3 tbsp. coconut flour

Directions:

1. Preheat the waffle iron.
2. In a small bowl, add water and chia seeds and soak for 5 minutes.
3. Mash together sunflower seed butter, lemon juice, vanilla, stevia, chia mixture, and avocado.
4. Mix together cinnamon, baking soda, and coconut flour.
5. Add wet ingredients to the dry ingredients and mix well.
6. Pour waffle mixture into the hot waffle iron and cook on each side for 3-5 minutes.
7. Serve and enjoy.

Cheese Almond Pancakes

Level of difficulty: 5

Preparation time: 10 minutes

Servings: 4

Calories: 271

Condiments: Cinnamon

Protein: 10.8 g

Fat: 25 g

Ingredients:

- 4 eggs
- 1/4 tsp cinnamon
- 1/2 cup cream cheese
- 1/2 cup almond flour
- 1 tbsp. butter, melted

Directions:

1. Add all ingredients into the blender and blend until combined.
2. Melt butter in a pan over medium heat.
3. Pour 3 tablespoons of batter per pancake and cook for 2 minutes on each side.
4. Serve and enjoy.

Vegetable Quiche

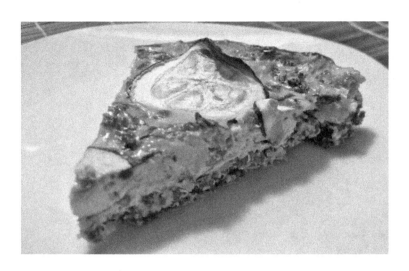

Level of difficulty: 5

Preparation time: 10 minutes

Servings: 6

Calories: 25

Condiments: Salt and Pepper

Protein: 22 g

Fat: 16.7 g

Ingredients:

- 8 eggs
- 1 onion, chopped
- 1 cup Parmesan cheese, grated
- 1 cup unsweetened coconut milk

- 1 cup tomatoes, chopped
- 1 cup zucchini, chopped
- 1 tbsp. butter
- 1/2 tsp pepper
- 1 tsp salt

Directions:

1. Preheat the oven to 400 F.
2. Melt butter in a pan over medium heat then add onion and sauté until onion soften.
3. Add tomatoes and zucchini to pan and sauté for 4 minutes.
4. Beat eggs with cheese, milk, pepper and salt in a bowl.
5. Pour egg mixture over vegetables and bake in oven for 30 minutes.
6. Slices and serve.

Pumpkin Muffins

Level of difficulty: 5

Preparation time: 10 minutes

Servings: 10

Calories: 150

Condiments: Salt

Protein: 5 g

Fat: 13 g

Ingredients:

- 4 eggs
- 1/2 cup pumpkin puree
- 1 tsp pumpkin pie spice
- 1/2 cup almond flour
- 1 tbsp. baking powder
- 1 tsp vanilla
- 1/3 cup coconut oil, melted
- 2/3 cup swerve
- 1/2 cup coconut flour
- 1/2 tsp sea salt

Directions:

1. Preheat the oven to 350 F.
2. In a large bowl, stir together coconut flour, pumpkin pie spice, baking powder, swerve, almond flour, and sea salt.
3. Stir in eggs, vanilla, coconut oil, and pumpkin puree until well combined.
4. Pour batter into the greased muffin tray and bake in oven for 25 minutes.
5. Serve and enjoy.

Cheesy Spinach Quiche

Level of difficulty: 5

Preparation time: 10 minutes

Servings: 6

Calories: 365

Condiments: Salt

Protein: 16.1 g

Fat: 31.5 g

Ingredients:

- 8 eggs
- 2 cups fresh spinach
- 1/2 cup feta cheese, crumbled
- 1/2 cup parmesan cheese, shredded
- 1/4 cup cheddar cheese, shredded
- 3 garlic cloves, minced
- 2 cups unsweetened almond milk
- 1/4 tsp salt

Directions:

1. In a large bowl, whisk together eggs and almond milk.
2. Add spinach, parmesan cheese, feta cheese, garlic, and salt and stir well to combine.
3. Spray crock pot with cooking spray.
4. Pour egg mixture into the crock pot.
5. Sprinkle shredded cheddar cheese over the top of egg mixture.
6. Cover and cook on low for 7 hours.

Kale and Walnuts

Level of difficulty: 5

Preparation time: 5 minutes

Servings: 4

Calories: 160

Condiments: Salt and Pepper

Protein: 5 g

Fat: 7 g

Ingredients:

- 3 garlic cloves
- 10 cups kale, roughly chopped.
- 1/3 cup parmesan, grated
- ½ cup almond milk
- ¼ cup walnuts, chopped.
- 1 tbsp. butter, melted
- ¼ tsp. nutmeg, ground
- Salt and black pepper to taste

Directions:

1. In a pan that fits the air fryer, combine all the ingredients, toss, introduce the pan in the machine, and cook at 360°F for 15 minutes.
2. Divide between plates and serve.

LUNCH

Baked Patties

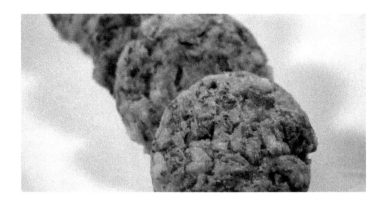

Level of difficulty: 8

Preparation time: 15 minutes

Servings: 4

Calories: 112

Condiments: Salt and Pepper

Protein: 16 g

Fat: 4.3 g

Ingredients:

- 1 lb. ground lamb
- 1 teaspoon ground coriander
- 1 teaspoon ground cumin
- ¼ cup fresh parsley, chopped
- ¼ cup onion, minced
- ¼ teaspoon cayenne pepper

- ½ teaspoon ground allspice
- 1 teaspoon ground cinnamon
- 1 tablespoon garlic, minced
- ¼ teaspoon pepper
- 1 teaspoon kosher salt

Directions:

1. Preheat the oven to 450 F.
2. Add all ingredients into the large bowl and mix until well combined.
3. Make small balls from meat mixture and place on a baking tray and lightly flatten the meatballs back on spoon.
4. Bake in preheated oven for 12-15 minutes.
5. Serve and enjoy.

Beef Ribeye Steak

Level of difficulty: 5

Preparation time: 5 minutes

Servings: 4

Calories: 293

Condiments: Salt and Pepper

Protein: 23 g

Fat: 22 g

Ingredients:

- 4 (8-ounce) ribeye steaks
- 1 tablespoon McCormick Grill Mates Montreal Steak Seasoning
- Salt
- Pepper

Directions:

1. Season the steaks with the steak seasoning and salt and pepper to taste. Place 2 steaks in the Cuisinart Air Fryer Oven. You can use an accessory grill pan, a layer rack, or the air fryer basket.
2. Cook for 4 minutes. Open the air fryer and flip the steaks.
3. Cook for an additional 4 to 5 minutes. Check for doneness to determine how much additional cook time is need. Remove the cooked steaks from the Cuisinart Air Fryer Oven, then repeat for the remaining 2 steaks.
4. Cool before serving.

Bacon Spaghetti Squash Carbonara

Level of difficulty: 5

Preparation time: 20 minutes

Servings: 4

Calories: 305

Condiments: Salt and Pepper

Protein: 18 g

Fat: 21 g

Ingredients:

- 1 small spaghetti squash
- 6 ounces' bacon (roughly chopped)
- 1 large tomato (sliced)
- 2 chives (chopped)
- 1 garlic clove (minced)
- 6 ounces' low-fat cottage cheese
- 1 cup Gouda cheese (grated)
- 2 tablespoons olive oil
- Salt and pepper, to taste

Directions:

1. Preheat the oven to 350°F.

2. Cut the squash spaghetti in half, brush with some olive oil and bake for 20–30 minutes, skin side up. Remove from the oven and remove the core with a fork, creating the spaghetti.

3. Heat one tablespoon of olive oil in a skillet. Cook the bacon for about 1 minute until crispy.

4. Quickly wipe out the pan with paper towels.

5. Heat another tablespoon of oil and sauté the garlic, tomato and chives for 2–3 minutes. Add the spaghetti and sauté for another 5 minutes, occasionally stirring to keep from burning.

6. Begin to add the cottage cheese, about 2 tablespoons at a time. If the sauce becomes thicken, add about a cup of water. The sauce should be creamy but not too runny or thick. Allow cooking for another 3 minutes.

7. Serve immediately.

Lean and Green Chicken Pesto Pasta

Level of difficulty: 5

Preparation time: 5 minutes

Servings: 1

Calories: 224

Condiments: Salt and Pepper

Protein: 20.5 g

Fat: 10 g

Ingredients:

- 3 cups of raw kale leaves
- 2 tbsp. of olive oil
- 2 cups of fresh basil
- 1/4 teaspoon salt
- 3 tbsp. lemon juice
- Three garlic cloves
- 2 cups of cooked chicken breast
- 1 cup of baby spinach
- 6 ounce of uncooked chicken pasta
- 3 ounces of diced fresh mozzarella
- Basil leaves or red pepper flakes to garnish

Directions:

1. Start by making the pesto, add the kale, lemon juice, basil, garlic cloves, olive oil, and salt to a blender and blend until its smooth.
2. Add salt and pepper to taste.
3. Cook the pasta and strain off the water. Reserve 1/4 cup of the liquid.
4. Get a bowl and mix everything, the cooked pasta, pesto, diced chicken, spinach, mozzarella, and the reserved pasta liquid.
5. Sprinkle the mixture with additional chopped basil or red paper flakes (optional).
6. Now your salad is ready. You may serve it warm or chilled. Also, it can be taken as a salad mix-ins or as a side dish. Leftovers should be stored in the refrigerator inside an air-tight container for 3-5 days.

Zucchini Egg Casserole

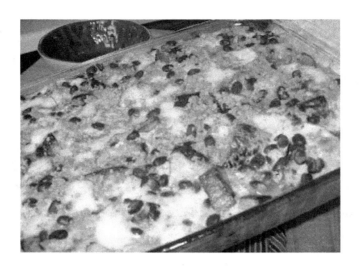

Level of difficulty: 5

Preparation time: 10 minutes

Servings: 8

Calories: 134

Condiments: Salt and Pepper

Protein: 8.8 g

Fat: 9.8 g

Ingredients:

- 10 eggs
- 3 cherry tomatoes, halved
- 1/2 cup mushrooms, sliced
- 1/3 cup ham, chopped

- 1 small zucchini, sliced into rounds
- 1/2 cup spinach
- 2/3 cup heavy cream
- Pepper
- Salt

Directions:

1. Preheat the oven to 350 F. Grease 9*13-inch pan and set aside.
2. In a large bowl, whisk eggs with heavy cream, pepper, and salt. Stir in tomatoes, mushrooms, ham, zucchini, and spinach.
3. Pour egg mixture in prepared pan and bake for 30-35 minutes.
4. Serve and enjoy.

Delicious Zucchini Quiche

Level of difficulty: 5

Preparation time: 10 minutes

Servings: 8

Calories: 288

Condiments: Salt

Protein: 11 g

Fat: 26.3 g

Ingredients

- 6 eggs
- 2 medium zucchinis, shredded
- 1/2 tsp. dried basil
- 2 garlic cloves, minced
- 1 tbsp. dry onion, minced
- 2 tbsp. parmesan cheese, grated
- 2 tbsp. fresh parsley, chopped
- 1/2 cup olive oil
- 1 cup cheddar cheese, shredded
- 1/4 cup coconut flour
- 3/4 cup almond flour
- 1/2 tsp. salt

Directions:

1. Preheat the oven to 350 F.

2. Grease 9-inch pie dish and set aside.

3. Squeeze out excess liquid from zucchini.

4. Add all ingredients into the large bowl and mix until well combined.

5. Pour into the prepared pie dish.

6. Bake in preheated oven for 45-60 minutes or until set.

7. Remove from the oven and let it cool completely.

8. Slice and serve.

Roasted Broccoli

Level of difficulty: 5

Preparation time: 10 minutes

Servings: 4

Calories: 205

Condiments: Salt and Pepper

Protein: 7.5 g

Fat: 16 g

Ingredients:

- 2 lbs broccoli, cut into florets
- 3 tbsp. olive oil
- 1 tbsp. lemon juice
- 1/4 cup parmesan cheese, grated
- ¼ cup almonds, sliced and toasted
- 3 garlic cloves, sliced
- ½ tsp red pepper flakes
- 1/4 tsp pepper
- 1/4 tsp salt

Directions:

1. Preheat the oven to 425 F.
2. Add broccoli, pepper, salt, garlic, and oil in large bowl and toss well.
3. Spread broccoli on baking tray and roast in for 20 minutes.
4. Add lemon juice, grated cheese, red pepper flakes and almonds over broccoli and toss well.
5. Serve and enjoy.

Stir Fried Broccoli with Mushroom

Level of difficulty: 5

Preparation time: 10 minutes

Servings: 4

Calories: 105

Condiments: Salt and Pepper

Protein: 5 g

Fat: 5 g

Ingredients:

- 2 cups broccoli, cut into florets
- 1 1/2 tsp fresh ginger, grated
- 1/4 tsp red pepper flakes
- 2 cups mushrooms, sliced
- 2 garlic cloves, minced
- 1 small onion, chopped
- 2 tbsp. balsamic vinegar
- 1/2 tbsp. sesame seeds
- 2 tbsp. soy sauce, low-sodium
- 1/4 cup cashews
- 1 medium carrot, shredded
- 3 tbsp. water

Directions:

1. Heat large pan over high heat.
2. Add broccoli, water, ginger, red pepper, mushrooms, garlic, and onion and cook until softened.
3. Add carrots, soy sauce, vinegar, and cashews. Stir well and simmer for 2 minutes.
4. Garnish with sesame seeds and serve

MID AFTERNOON

Sausage and Cheese Dip

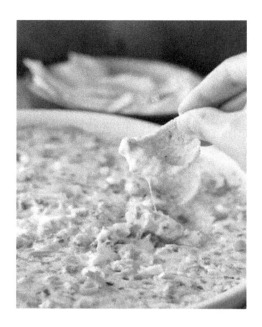

Level of difficulty: 5

Preparation time: 10 minutes

Servings: 28

Calories: 132

Condiments: Salt and Pepper

Protein: 6.79 g

Fat: 9.58 g

Ingredients:

- 8 ounces cream cheese
- A pinch of salt and black pepper
- 16 ounces sour cream
- 8 ounces pepper jack cheese, chopped
- 15 ounces canned tomatoes mixed with habaneros
- 1-pound Italian sausage, ground
- ¼ cup green onions, chopped

Directions:

1. Heat a pan over medium heat, add sausage, stir and cook until it browns.
2. Add tomatoes mix, stir and cook for 4 minutes more.
3. Add a pinch of salt, pepper, and the green onions, stir and cook for 4 minutes.
4. Spread pepper jack cheese on the bottom of your slow cooker.
5. Add cream cheese, sausage mix, sour cream, cover and cook on High for 2 hours.
6. Uncover your slow cooker, stir dip, transfer to a bowl, and serve.
7. Enjoy!

Tasty Onion and Cauliflower Dip

Level of difficulty: 5

Preparation time: 20 minutes

Servings: 24

Calories: 40

Condiments: Salt and Pepper

Protein: 1.32 g

Fat: 3.31 g

Ingredients:

- 1 and ½ cups chicken stock
- 1 cauliflower head, florets separated
- ¼ cup mayonnaise
- ½ cup yellow onion, chopped
- ¾ cup cream cheese
- ½ teaspoon chili powder
- ½ teaspoon cumin, ground
- ½ teaspoon garlic powder
- Salt and black pepper to the taste

Directions:

1. Put the stock in a pot, add cauliflower and onion, heat up over medium heat, and cook for 30 minutes.
2. Add chili powder, salt, pepper, cumin, and garlic powder and stir.
3. Also, add cream cheese and stir a bit until it melts.
4. Blend using an immersion blender and mix with the mayo.
5. Transfer to a bowl and keep in the fridge for 2 hours before you serve it.
6. Enjoy!

Pesto Crackers

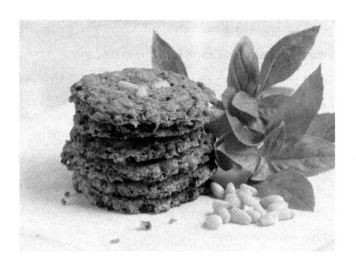

Level of difficulty: 5

Preparation time: 10 minutes

Servings: 6

Calories: 9

Condiments: Cayenne Pepper

Protein: 0.41 g

Fat: 0.14 g

Ingredients:

- ½ teaspoon baking powder
- Salt and black pepper to the taste
- 1 and ¼ cups almond flour

- ¼ teaspoon basil, dried 1 garlic clove, minced
- 2 tablespoons basil pesto
- A pinch of cayenne pepper
- 3 tablespoons ghee

Directions:

1. In a bowl, mix salt, pepper, baking powder, and almond flour.
2. Add garlic, cayenne, and basil and stir.
3. Add pesto and whisk.
4. Also, add ghee and mix your dough with your finger.
5. Spread this dough on a lined baking sheet, introduce in the oven at 325 degrees F and bake for 17 minutes.
6. Leave aside to cool down, cut your crackers, and serve them as a snack.
7. Enjoy!

Pumpkin Muffins

Level of difficulty: 5

Preparation time: 15 minutes

Servings: 18

Calories: 65

Condiments: Salt

Protein: 2.82 g

Fat: 5.42 g

Ingredients:

- ¼ cup sunflower seed butter
- ¾ cup pumpkin puree
- 2 tablespoons flaxseed meal
- ¼ cup coconut flour
- ½ cup erythritol
- ½ teaspoon nutmeg, ground
- 1 teaspoon cinnamon, ground
- ½ teaspoon baking soda
- 1 egg ½ teaspoon baking powder
- A pinch of salt

Directions:

1. In a bowl, mix butter with pumpkin puree and egg and blend well.
2. Add flaxseed meal, coconut flour, erythritol, baking soda, baking powder, nutmeg, cinnamon, and a pinch of salt and stir well.
3. Spoon this into a greased muffin pan, introduce in the oven at 350 degrees F and bake for 15 minutes.
4. Leave muffins to cool down and serve them as a snack.
5. Enjoy!

Bacon Cheeseburger

Level of difficulty: 5

Preparation time: 10 minutes

Servings: 4

Calories: 30

Condiments: Salt

Protein: 15 g

Fat: 14 g

Ingredients:

- 1 lb. lean ground beef
- 1/4 cup chopped yellow onion
- 1 clove garlic, minced
- 1 tbsp. yellow mustard
- 1 tbsp. Worcestershire sauce
- 1/2 tsp. salt
- Cooking spray
- 4 ultra-thin slices cheddar cheese, cut into 6 equal-sized rectangular pieces
- 3 pieces of turkey bacon, each cut into 8 evenly-sized rectangular pieces
- 24 dill pickle chips
- 4-6 green leaf

- Lettuce leaves, torn into 24 small square-shaped pieces
- 12 cherry tomatoes, sliced in half

Directions:

1. Pre-heat oven to 400°F.
2. Combine the garlic, salt, onion, Worcestershire sauce, and beef in a medium-sized bowl, and mix well.
3. Form mixture into 24 small meatballs.
4. Put meatballs onto a foil-lined baking sheet and cook for 12-15 minutes.
5. Leave oven on.
6. Top every meatball with a piece of cheese, then go back to the oven until cheese melts for about 2 to 3 minutes.
7. Let meatballs cool.
8. To assemble bites: on a toothpick layer a cheese-covered meatball, piece of bacon, piece of lettuce, pickle chip, and a tomato half.

DINNER

Arugula Lentil Salad

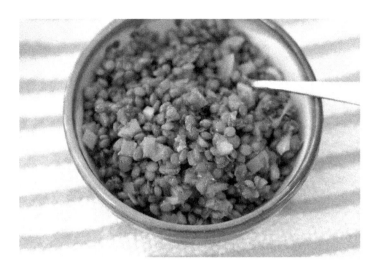

Level of difficulty: 3

Preparation time: 20 minutes

Servings: 1

Calories: 319

Condiments: Salt and Pepper

Protein: 13.25 g

Fat: 16.06 g

Ingredients:

- 3 cups Arugula, fresh

- 1/2 Avocado, ripe

- 1 stalk Celery

- 2 cloves Garlic
- 1/2 Lemon
- 1 cup Lentils, green
- 1 cup Tomatoes
- Baking & Spices
- 1 Pepper, ground fresh
- 1 Salt
- Oils & Vinegars
- 1 Olive oil, extra virgin
- Dairy
- 1 Goat cheese

Directions:

1. Boil water and add lentils. Cook for 20 minutes until lentils are tender.
2. Place olive oil, parsley, pepper, salt, and garlic in a blender and puree.
3. Mix cooked lentils, avocado, celery, arugula, lemon juice, and olive oil mixture in a saucepan and heat for 5 minutes.
4. Place a large scoop of salad in a bowl, crumble goat cheese on the salad, and drizzle with vinegar.

Creamy Corn Soup

Level of difficulty: 3

Preparation time: 10 minutes

Servings: 4

Calories: 95

Condiments: Salt and Pepper

Protein: 1.59 g

Fat: 15.61 g

Ingredients:

- One-half onion, chopped
- 1 clove garlic, minced
- One-fourth cup chopped fresh parsley
- 1 tablespoon margarine
- 3 tablespoons all-purpose flour
- 2 and one-half cups milk
- 1 cup chicken broth
- 2 (12 ounce) cans whole kernel corn
- 2 and one-half tablespoons cream cheese
- 1 teaspoon garlic salt
- 1 teaspoon ground black pepper
- ground cayenne pepper to taste

Directions:

1. Heat olive oil in a large saucepan. Sauté onion and garlic over medium heat until tender. Mix onion, garlic, parsley, and any other assorted vegetables.
2. Sauté this mixture for three minutes stirring for even cooking.
3. In a separate saucepan, melt the margarine. Stir in flour. Slowly stir in the cheese. Cook, stirring constantly, over medium heat for about three minutes.
4. Stir for about a minute over medium-low heat.
5. Add broth by gradually add milk for a smooth mixture. Cook over medium heat, stirring frequently until the mixture thickens.
6. Add corn and heat through.
7. Add sifted salt, pepper, and garlic salt.
8. Add the cheese mixture. Cook and stir until cheese melts.
9. Garnish with fresh parsley and paprika.

Eggplant Curry

Level of difficulty: 3

Preparation time: 20 minutes

Servings: 8

Calories: 95

Condiments: Garlic powder

Protein: 1.59 g

Fat: 15.61 g

Ingredients:

- Broccoli soup (1.0 Envelope)

- Baking Powder (Low Sodium) (0.5 tsp)

- Garlic Powder (1.0 tsp)

- Water (3.0 tbsp.)

- Parmesan cheese - Reduced-fat (2.0 tbsp.)

- Eggplant - Sliced (1.5 cups)

- Egg Beaters - Original (0.25 cup)

- Walden Farms Marinara Sauce (0.25 cup)

- Garlic Powder (1.0 tsp)

- 2% Reduced fat Mozzarella Cheese (3.5 oz.)

Directions:

1. Nuke broccoli soup for 2 minutes in the microwave. Add water, baking powder, garlic powder, and parmesan cheese. Mix thoroughly until the water is creamy and powder is dissolved. Set aside.
2. Take cupcake pan and line with cups. Make sure the pan is sprayed with nonstick spray.
3. Place a spoonful of broccoli mix into each of the 12 cups. Layer eggplant and egg beaters over the top. Pour marinara sauce over eggplant. Sprinkle garlic powder and sprinkle mozzarella cheese on top.
4. Bake in a 375-degree oven for 25 minutes.

Asian Cabbage Rice

Level of difficulty: 3

Preparation time: 10 minutes

Servings: 2

Calories: 95

Condiments: Stacey Hawkins Wok on or Stacey Hawkins Tasty Thai Seasoning

Protein: 1.59 g

Fat: 15.61 g

Ingredients:

- 4 cup cabbage, minced into a rice-like texture (can also use cabbage slaw blend- watch carrots)
- 1 T Stacey Hawkins Wok on or Stacey Hawkins Tasty Thai Seasoning
- 1/2 cup water
- fresh lime slice
- fresh cilantro & green onion (optional)

Directions:

1. Heat Wok on high heat.
2. Add 1 tablespoon oil and stir-fry until softened, approx. 2 minutes.

3. Pour in water and cover.

4. Stir-fry until cooked, approx. 1 minute.

5. Remove wok from heat. Stir in cabbage.

6. Cover & cook for 1 minute.

7. Add seasoning to taste.

8. Cut a lime into wedges.

9. Garnish with fresh cilantro and green onion.

Note: Can be to serve over hot or cold noodles or zucchini pasta.

African Peanut Soup

Level of difficulty: 3

Preparation time: 15 minutes

Servings: 10

Calories: 95

Condiments: Chili powder

Protein: 1.59 g

Fat: 15.61 g

Ingredients:

- 2 tablespoons olive oil
- 2 medium onions, chopped
- 2 large red bell peppers, chopped
- 4 cloves garlic, minced
- 1 (28 ounces) can crushed tomatoes, with liquid
- 8 cups vegetable broth or stock
- One-fourth teaspoon pepper
- One-fourth teaspoon chili powder
- Two-thirds cup extra crunchy peanut butter
- One-half cup uncooked brown rice

Directions:

1. Heat the oil in a large pot. Sauté the onions, red bell peppers, and garlic. Cook for 5 minutes.
2. Add the crushed tomatoes and vegetable broth. Bring to a boil. Reduce heat. Simmer for about 20 minutes.
3. Add pepper and chili powder. Stir in the peanut butter and brown rice.
4. Cover and cook over low heat for about 30 minutes.

Tip: Serve the soup with a slice of lemon.

Sweet Potato Soup

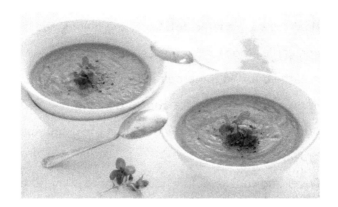

Level of difficulty: 3

Preparation time: 20 minutes

Servings: 3-4

Calories: 95

Condiments: Pepper and Chili Flakes

Protein: 1.59 g

Fat: 15.61 g

Ingredients:

- 1 tbsp. olive oil
- 1 onion, roughly chopped
- 2 large carrots, peeled and roughly chopped
- 4cm/1½ inches fresh root ginger, finely chopped
- 1 garlic clove, crushed

- ½ tsp dried red chili flakes
- 700g/1lb 10oz sweet potatoes, peeled and cubed
- 1.2 liters/2 pints vegetable stock
- salt and freshly ground black pepper

Directions:

1. Heat the oil in a large saucepan over medium-high heat. Sauté the leeks, onion, and carrots until slightly softened, 5 minutes.
2. Add the ginger, garlic, and chili flakes and cook for 1 to 2 minutes.
3. Stir in the sweet potato and fry until it begins to soften. Add the stock, bring to the boil. Reduce the heat and simmer for about 15 minutes, or until the sweet potato is cooked through.
4. Pour the soup into a blender and blend until smooth.
5. Season with salt and pepper to taste. Serve hot.

Roasted Garlic Wilted Spinach

Level of difficulty: 3

Preparation time: 10 minutes

Servings: 4

Calories: 95

Condiments: feta cheese

Protein: 1.59 g

Fat: 15.61 g

Ingredients:

- 6 cups spinach
- 1 tsp olive oil
- 5 cloves garlic; or to taste
- 1/8 cup feta cheese
- 4 tabs chopped walnuts

Directions:

1. Preheat oven to 375F.
2. Parboil spinach in a pot of boiling water for 6 minutes or till wilted and soft. Drain and pat dry with a paper towel
3. In a hot skillet, drop in the garlic, and sauté till fragrant.
4. Mix in spinach and sauté on medium heat till wilted.

5. Remove to a plate and keep warm.

6. Spray with oil and layout in a baking sheet in a single layer.

7. Roast till golden brown.

8. Top with feta cheese and walnuts and serve immediately.

Baba Ganoush

Level of difficulty: 3

Preparation time: 20 minutes

Servings: 6

Calories: 95

Condiments: Paprika

Protein: 1.59 g

Fat: 15.61 g

Cooking time: 35 minutes

Ingredients:

- 2 pounds Italian eggplants (about 2 small-to-medium eggplants*)
- 2 medium cloves of garlic, pressed or minced
- 2 tablespoons lemon juice, more if necessary
- ¼ cup tahini
- One-third cup extra-virgin olive oil, plus more for brushing the eggplant and garnish
- 2 tablespoons chopped fresh flat-leaf parsley, plus extra for garnish
- Three-fourth teaspoon salt, to taste
- ¼ teaspoon ground cumin
- Pinch of smoked paprika, for garnish

Serving suggestions: warmed or toasted pita wedges, carrot sticks, bell pepper strips, cucumber slices, etc.

Directions:

1. With a sharp knife, cut the eggplants half lengthwise, removing the stem and the seed pod.
2. Place the halves cut-side down on a baking sheet.
3. Bake for about 40 minutes, until the flesh is very soft.
4. When they're cool enough to handle, scoop out the flesh and transfer to a bowl.
5. Add to the bowl the garlic, lemon juice, tahini, one-third cup oil, parsley, salt, and cumin.
6. Use a fork to mash and purée until the mixture is very smooth.
7. Adjust the seasonings to your taste.
8. Place in a serving bowl, drizzle with a little extra-virgin olive oil and sprinkle with a touch of paprika and fresh parsley.
9. Give it a good stir and adjust the seasoning again if need be.
10. Serve with wedges of toasted pita bread, carrot sticks, bell pepper strips, cucumber slices, or other good things in life.

Roasted Garlic Zoodles

Level of difficulty: 3

Preparation time: 15 minutes

Servings: 4

Calories: 95

Condiments: Zucchini

Protein: 1.59 g

Fat: 15.61 g

Ingredients:

- 10 ounces grape tomatoes
- 1 tablespoon grapeseed oil (or any neutral-flavored cooking oil you have on hand)
- 1 teaspoon dried oregano
- Salt to taste
- 2 pounds zucchini, spiralized
- 2 tablespoons fresh lemon juice
- 2 tablespoons extra-virgin olive oil
- 1 teaspoon lemon zest
- 1 large clove garlic, minced
- 3 tablespoons toasted pine nuts

Directions:

1. Preheat oven to 400ºF. In a large bowl, toss the tomatoes with the oil, oregano, and salt pinch. Transfer to a baking sheet and roast until charred in spots, about 10 minutes.
2. Cook the zoodles in a pot of boiling water until just tender, about 2 minutes, depending on the width of your zoodles.
3. Drain and immediately transfer to a large bowl of ice water to shock them and stop the cooking process. Drain the zoodles again and place them in a large bowl along with the lemon juice (calms the bitter taste from the zucchini), the olive oil, lemon zest, and garlic.
4. Toss to coat. Remove the tomatoes from the oven and let cool slightly about 5 minutes. Roughly chop and add them to the bowl along with the pine nuts, sprinkle with salt, and toss again to combine. Serve immediately.

Nutty Charred Broccoli

Level of difficulty: 3

Preparation time: 10 minutes

Servings: 2

Calories: 95

Condiments: Stacey Hawkins Dash Desperation Seasoning

Protein: 1.59 g

Fat: 15.61 g

Preparation time: 10 minutes

Cooking time: 15 minutes

Servings: 4

Ingredients:

- 4 teaspoons fresh chopped garlic and oil
- 4 C broccoli florets, cut into approx. 1pieces
- 1 teaspoon capfuls Stacey Hawkins Dash of Desperation Seasoning.

Directions:

1. In a large saucepan, heat oil and add garlic. Cook on med-high 4 mins, stirring often.

2. add broccoli and Stacey Hawkins dash of desperation seasoning, cookout of cold on med-high another 8 mins stirring well.
3. turn heat to med and cook another 10 mins till nice and brown and tender.
4. serve hot or cool & store for future use. Enjoy

EVENING

Grilled Mahi Mahi with Jicama Slaw

Level of difficulty: 5

Preparation time: 20 minutes

Servings: 4

Calories: 288

Condiments: Salt and Pepper

Protein: 12.5 g

Fat: 10.2 g

Ingredients:

- 1 teaspoon each for pepper and salt, divided
- 1 tablespoon of lime juice, divided
- 2 tablespoon + 2 teaspoons of extra virgin olive oil
- 4 raw mahi-mahi fillets, which should be about 8 oz. each
- ½ cucumber which should be thinly cut into long strips like matchsticks (it should yield about 1 cup)
- 1 jicama, which should be thinly cut into long strips like matchsticks (it should yield about 3 cups)
- 1 cup of alfalfa sprouts
- 2 cups of coarsely chopped watercress

Directions:

1. Combine ½ teaspoon of both pepper and salt, 1 teaspoon of lime juice, and 2 teaspoons of oil in a small bowl. Then brush the mahi-mahi fillets all through with the olive oil mixture.

2. Grill the mahi-mahi on medium-high heat until it becomes done in about 5 minutes, turn it to the other side, and let it be done for about 5 minutes. (You will have an internal temperature of about 1450F).

3. For the slaw, combine the watercress, cucumber, jicama, and alfalfa sprouts in a bowl. Now combine ½ teaspoon of both pepper and salt, 2 teaspoons of lime juice, and 2 tablespoons of extra virgin oil in a small bowl. Drizzle it over slaw and toss together to combine.

Rosemary Cauliflower Rolls

Level of difficulty: 5

Preparation time: 10 minutes

Servings: 3

Calories: 288

Condiments: Salt

Protein: 12.5 g

Fat: 10.2 g

Ingredients:

- 1/3 cup of almond flour
- 4 cups of riced cauliflower
- 1/3 cup of reduced-fat, shredded mozzarella or cheddar cheese
- 2 eggs
- 2 tablespoons of fresh rosemary, finely chopped
- ½ teaspoon of salt

Directions:

1. Preheat your oven to 4000F
2. Combine all the listed ingredients in a medium-sized bowl
3. Scoop cauliflower mixture into 12 evenly-sized rolls/biscuits onto a lightly-greased and foil-lined baking sheet.

4. Bake until it turns golden brown, which should be achieved in about 30 minutes.
5. Note: if you want to have the outside of the rolls/biscuits crisp, then broil for some minutes before serving.

Beef Stroganoff

Level of difficulty: 5

Preparation time: 10 minutes

Servings: 2

Calories: 470

Condiments: Salt and Pepper

Protein: 49 g

Fat: 25 g

Ingredients:

- 1/2 lb. beef stew meat
- 10 oz. mushroom soup, homemade
- 1 medium onion, chopped
- 1/2 cup sour cream
- oz. mushrooms, sliced
- Pepper and salt

Directions:

1. Add all ingredients except sour cream into the crock pot and mix well.
2. Cover and cook on low heat for 8 hours.
3. Add sour cream and stir well.
4. Serve and enjoy.

Lemon Beef

Level of difficulty: 4

Preparation time: 10 minutes

Servings: 4

Calories: 355

Condiments: Salt and Chili Powder

Protein: 35.5 g

Fat: 16.8 g

Ingredients:

- 1 lb. beef chuck roast
- 1 fresh lime juice
- 1 garlic clove, crushed
- 1 teaspoon chili powder
- 2 cups lemon-lime soda
- 1/2 teaspoon salt

Directions:

1. Place beef chuck roast into the slow cooker.
2. Season roast with garlic, chili powder, and salt.
3. Pour lemon-lime soda over the roast.
4. Cover slow cooker and cook on low for 6 hours. Shred the meat using fork.
5. Add lime juice over shredded roast and serve.

Herb Pork Roast

Level of difficulty: 5

Preparation time: 10 minutes

Servings: 10

Calories: 327

Condiments: Salt

Protein: 59 g

Fat: 8 g

Ingredients:

- 5 lbs. pork roast, boneless or bone-in
- 1 tablespoon dry herb mix
- 4 garlic cloves, cut into slivers
- 1 tablespoon salt

Directions:

1. Using a knife make small cuts all over meat then insert garlic slivers into the cuts.
2. In a small bowl, mix Italian herb mix and salt and rub all over pork roast.
3. Place pork roast in the crock pot.

4. Cover and cook on low heat for 14 hours.

5. Extract meat from crock pot and shred using a fork.

6. Serve and enjoy.

Greek Beef Roast

Level of difficulty: 6

Preparation time: 10 minutes

Servings: 6

Calories: 231

Condiments: Salt and Pepper

Protein: 35 g

Fat: 6 g

Ingredients:

- 2 lbs. lean top round beef roast
- 1 tablespoon Italian seasoning
- 6 garlic cloves, minced
- 1 onion, sliced
- 2 cups beef broth
- ½ cup red wine
- 1 teaspoon red pepper flakes
- Pepper
- Salt

Directions:

1. Season meat with pepper and salt and place into the crock pot.
2. Pour remaining ingredients over meat.
3. Cover and cook on low heat for 8 hours.
4. Shred the meat using fork.
5. Serve and enjoy.

Tomato Pork Chops

Level of difficulty: 5

Preparation time: 10 minutes

Servings: 4

Calories: 325

Condiments: Kosher Salt and Pepper

Protein: 20 g

Fat: 23.4 g

Ingredients:

- 4 pork chops, bone-in
- 1 tablespoon garlic, minced
- ½ small onion, chopped
- 6 oz. can tomato paste
- 1 bell pepper, chopped
- ¼ teaspoon red pepper flakes
- 1 teaspoon Worcestershire sauce
- 1 tablespoon dried Italian seasoning
- 14.5 oz. can tomato, diced
- 2 teaspoon olive oil
- ¼ teaspoon pepper
- 1 teaspoon kosher salt

Directions:

1. Heat oil in a pan over heat.
2. Season pork chops with pepper and salt.
3. Sear pork chops in pan until brown from both the sides.
4. Transfer pork chops into the crock pot.
5. Add remaining ingredients over pork chops.
6. Cover and cook on low heat for 6 hours.
7. Serve and enjoy.

Greek Pork Chops

Level of difficulty: 5

Preparation time: 10 minutes

Servings: 8

Calories: 324

Condiments: Salt and Pepper

Protein: 18 g

Fat: 26.5 g

Ingredients:

- 8 pork chops, boneless
- 4 teaspoon dried oregano
- 2 tablespoon Worcestershire sauce
- 3 tablespoon fresh lemon juice
- ¼ cup olive oil
- 1 teaspoon ground mustard
- 2 teaspoon garlic powder
- 2 teaspoon onion powder
- Pepper
- Salt

Directions:

- Whisk together oil, garlic powder, onion powder, oregano, Worcestershire sauce, lemon juice, mustard, pepper, and salt.
- Place pork chops in a dish then pour marinade over pork chops and coat well. Place in refrigerator overnight.
- Preheat the grill.
- Place pork chops on the grill and cook for 3-4 minutes on each side.
- Serve and enjoy.

Tender Lamb Chops

Level of difficulty: 7

Preparation time: 10 minutes

Servings: 8

Calories: 40

Condiments: Salt and Pepper

Protein: 3.4 g

Fat: 1.9 g

Ingredients:

- 8 lamb chops
- ½ teaspoon dried thyme
- 1 onion, sliced
- 1 teaspoon dried oregano
- 2 garlic cloves, minced
- Pepper and salt

Directions:

1. Add sliced onion into the slow cooker.
2. Combine thyme, oregano, pepper, and salt. Rub over lamb chops.
3. Place lamb chops in slow cooker and top with garlic.
4. Pour ¼ cup water around the lamb chops.
5. Cover and cook on low heat for 6 hours.
6. Serve and enjoy.

Smoky Pork & Cabbage

Level of difficulty: 8

Preparation time: 10 minutes

Servings: 6

Calories: 484

Condiments: Salt

Protein: 66 g

Fat: 21.5 g

Ingredients:

- 3 lbs. pork roast
- 1/2 cabbage head, chopped
- 1 cup water
- 1/3 cup liquid smoke
- 1 tablespoon kosher salt

Directions:

1. Rub pork with kosher salt and place into the crock pot.
2. Pour liquid smoke over the pork. Add water.
3. Cover and cook on low heat for 7 hours.

4. Remove pork from crock pot and add cabbage in the bottom of crock pot.
5. Place pork on top of the cabbage.
6. Cover again and cook for 1 more hour.
7. Shred pork with a fork and serve.

Seasoned Pork Chops

Level of difficulty: 6

Preparation time: 10 minutes

Servings: 4

Calories: 386

Condiments: Salt and Pepper

Protein: 20 g

Fat: 32.9 g

Ingredients:

- 4 pork chops
- 2 garlic cloves, minced
- 1 cup chicken broth
- 1 tablespoon poultry seasoning
- 1/4 cup olive oil
- Pepper and salt

Directions:

1. In a bowl, whisk together olive oil, poultry seasoning, garlic, broth, pepper, and salt.

2. Pour olive oil mixture into the slow cooker then place pork chops to the crock pot.
3. Cover and cook on high heat for 4 hours.
4. Serve and enjoy.

Beef Stroganoff

Level of difficulty: 7

Preparation time: 10 minutes

Servings: 2

Calories: 470

Condiments: Salt and Pepper

Protein: 49 g

Fat: 25 g

Ingredients:

- 1/2 lb. beef stew meat
- 10 oz. mushroom soup, homemade
- 1 medium onion, chopped
- 1/2 cup sour cream
- oz. mushrooms, sliced
- Pepper and salt

Directions:

1. Add all ingredients except sour cream into the crock pot and mix well.
2. Cover and cook on low heat for 8 hours.
3. Add sour cream and stir well.
4. Serve and enjoy.

CONCLUSION

Thank you for reading all this book!

We hope that with the information you have learned, you will soon gain a healthier and happier lifestyle. You can enjoy gaining healthier bodies, lower blood pressure, reduced cholesterol, and healthier blood sugar. By combining this book and some consultation, you can live better and longer.

Best wishes!

Melissa Roberts

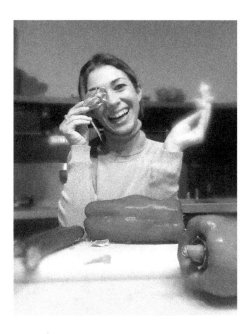

Melissa Roberts came from a humble beginning. Melissa gets satisfaction from helping individuals and families achieve their nutrition and health goals. She is passionate about her faith, family, friends, food, and fitness. In her work, Melissa focuses on simplifying science and empowering people to make small changes that leads to better health. She strives to be clear and concise. She is always working to find a bit of balance in her own life.

9 781801 858342